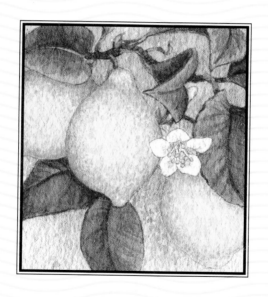

REFRESH YOUR ENERGY

INVIGORATING CITRUS

PUBLICATIONS INTERNATIONAL, LTD.

Louis Weber, C.E.O.
Publications International, Ltd.
7373 North Cicero Avenue
Lincolnwood, Illinois 60646

Permissions never granted for commercial purposes.

Manufactured in China.

8 7 6 5 4 3 2 1

ISBN: 0-7853-3414-9

Dawn Baumann Brunke has a degree in massage therapy from the Potomac Institute of Myotherapy and practices aromatherapy. She is editor of *Alaska Wellness* magazine and has authored many articles on holistic healing. Ms. Brunke wrote the introduction and profile text of this publication.

Margaret Anne Huffman is an award-winning writer and journalist. She has authored and co-authored inspirational titles including *Second Wind* and *Simple Wisdom*. She has also contributed to *Graces, Family Celebrations*, and *365 Daily Meditations for Women*. Ms. Huffman's work appears on pages 29, 36, 37, 38, 45, and 52.

Laurel Kallenbach is a freelance writer and poet. She has a master of arts degree in creative writing from Syracuse University and is former senior editor of *Delicious!* magazine. Ms. Kallenbach's work appears on pages 33, 34, 42, and 55.

Katherine Lyons is a writing professional and poet. She is founder of "The Society for Ladies Who Laugh Out Loud," a national network of women gathering to rekindle energy, perspective, a sense of humor, and positive focus. Ms. Lyon's work appears on pages 54 and 58.

Other material compiled by:
Helen H. Moore and Kelly Boyer Sagert

Note: This book does not constitute the practice of medicine. If you have any health questions or concerns, the publisher suggests you consult your doctor.

Aromatherapy:

An Introduction

How easy it is to become lost in the intoxicating fragrance of a flower garden, the pungent 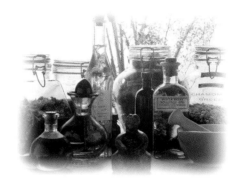 awakening of spices and dried herbs, the crisp burst of scent from a freshly peeled orange, or the sweet intensity of a newly bloomed rose. Aroma has the power to inspire, sedate, energize, and entice.

Aroma is also a link to other times and places. The sharp, earthy smell of burning leaves recalls dis-

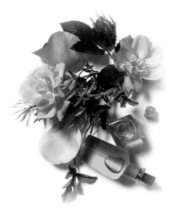

tant autumns; the aroma of gingerbread cookies conjures childhood memories; and the lingering perfume of a lover's scent summons the warm clasp of a close embrace.

Aroma means scent, but it has powers beyond those that arouse or arrest the senses. Within the fragrances of aromatic plants are substances that improve health, promote healing, and support your general well-being. These substances are found in the plant's essential oils, which are responsible for its unique fragrance as well as its healing benefits.

But aromatherapy doesn't work by the sense of smell alone. Essential oils can be used topically, taking direct action on surrounding tissues and entering the bloodstream to be carried throughout the body.

The modern world has newly discovered the enchanting magic of aroma as well as the potent healing gifts contained in essential oils. These gifts, though, have been used by mankind at least since biblical times, and probably before. Today we understand why and how essential oils treat psychological and physical illness. In ancient times, people just knew that they worked.

THE ANCIENT MEANING AND USE OF SCENT

Mysterious, invisible, and deeply moving, aroma was long believed to hold the soul of a plant, to be the essence of the divine. The Egyptians believed the

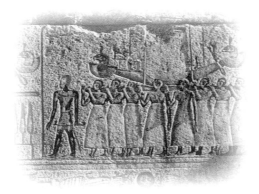

fleeting scent of a plant was a metaphor for the human soul. Ancient peoples believed deities would find prayers more pleasing when sweetly scented, and so the musky wisps of incense were used in nearly every culture to carry prayers heavenward. The ancients surrounded themselves with the richness of aroma, believing that as scented air entered their lungs and pores, a link was forged to the divine. In ancient Greece, oracles inhaled incense scented with bay leaves to inspire their visions, and Tibetan women captured aromatic clouds of cedar smoke to propel them into prophecy. Purifiers of body and soul, fragrant billows of smoke were also used to induce tranquility, insight, intoxication, and inner peace.

Ancient peoples also learned that heated animal fats could absorb the aromatic properties of fragrant flowers and leaves. When cooled, such concoctions were found to help heal wounds, soothe sore muscles, protect skin from the elements, and add a scent of mystery and allure to the wearer. It was later discovered that fragrance could be held in water as well, either to be ingested as a tonic or applied as scent to the skin and hair.

The Egyptians were famous for their scented oils. So masterfully did they blend essential oils that calcite pots once filled with their scented creations still held a faint aroma when the tomb of King Tutankhamen was opened 3,000 years later. The Romans bathed in fragrance, while the Greeks generously applied scented oils to their bodies. The East Indians turned the use of scent into a sensual art form. Women anointed their glistening, freshly bathed bodies with jasmine, sweet patchouli, amber, musk, sandalwood, and saffron. Each part of the body held a different scent, an aromatic garden of earthly delights.

The bewitching aspects of aroma are as old as the entanglement of love and power. Cleopatra lured Mark Anthony as her slaves burned incense and fanned the smoke into the sails of her ship. When the Queen of Sheba made her famous visit to King Solomon, it was to discuss the trading of fragrant resins. Delicately scented smoke was used to perfume a woman's hair in ancient Japan, and geishas measured their customer's stay by the number of incense sticks that were burned.

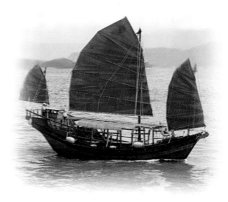

Ancient Athens was famous for merchants selling enticingly scented body oils, musks, aromatic perfumes, and disks of fragrant incense. The Phoenicians traded exotic wares of Chinese camphor, Indian cinnamon, and sandalwood. Aromatics merchants from India and Persia carried jasmine-scented sesame oil to China, while rosewater was mixed into the mortar used to build sacred mosques in the East. So was the world once connected by the pervasive and persuasive power of fragrance.

Aromatherapy Today

Today, aromatherapy has come of age. Offering not only sensual pleasure but a fragrant cure, essential oils are once again being used for their health benefits.

Enter, then, the provocative world of aroma with its incredible diversity of scent, from the seductive richness of jasmine to the sweet gentleness of lavender, from the tangy scent of citrus to the floral purity of rose. Whether you choose a scent to invigorate and exhilarate or refresh and soothe, aromatherapy is an exquisite journey into body, mind, and soul.

CITRUS

With a brisk tang, the scent of citrus is distinctively clean and delightfully invigorating. The 16-member citrus family includes the familiar lime, lemon, orange, grapefruit, and mandarin, as well as the less familiar bergamot. Although not entirely interchangeable, citrus family members all share some common attributes. They have a bright, fresh fragrance that is both revitalizing and uplifting. And several of the essential oils produced from this family are useful as disinfectants.

The bright, gleefully yellow lemon typifies the qualities of the citrus family. As its cheerful color implies, lemon is an antidepressant. Just a whiff of lemon essential oil can help dissipate mental fatigue, raise your spirits, and increase confidence. Lemon's lively fragrance improves concentration and increases alertness, relaxes brain waves, and calms the nerves. Inhaling the vitalizing scent of lemon, then, is excellent preparation for making difficult or complex decisions.

Lemon has a truly impressive range of therapeutic properties. It is both antibacterial and antiviral and is wonderfully suited to diffusion, helping to purify the air. It is often vaporized in sickrooms to renew stale air and kill germs. Like most citrus oils, the energizing scent of lemon instantly refreshes a room. For that reason, it is used in a vast number of household cleaning products. Lemon essential oil also increases the activity of the immune system, supporting our body's efforts to fight infection.

The aroma of lemon helps clear the head not just psychologically but of colds and fever as well. For many centuries a hot drink of honey, brandy, and lemon fruit or juice and peel has been used to sooth sore throats and coughs. Lemon essential oil is also a major ingredient in many commercial beverages, foods, and pharmaceuticals.

Early forms of the lemon are believed to have originated in China and other parts of Asia. Arabian merchants gathered loads of the lovely lemons and carried them to Italy and the Mediterranean, where

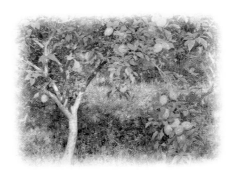 lemon trees are still cultivated today. Lemon trees develop heartily and with optimism, for a single lemon tree can produce up to 1,500 lemons a year. Sensitive to cold temperatures and high humidity, lemons fare best in arid, subtropical climates, where they grow in bright, sunny, fragrant orchards.

Because of its sharp and invigorating scent, lemon was used in ancient times to perfume clothes and repel insects. In the seventeenth century, lemon was noted to be a blood cleanser. It was not until much later, however, that lemon's medicinal value was discovered. Because of its vitamin C content, lemon was found to counteract scurvy. When great quantities of it (and other citrus fruits) were issued for lengthy sea voyages by the British Navy, lemon became renowned as a restorative healer. In time, the lemon was discovered to possess many other healing properties and was eventually proclaimed a universal remedy.

A few drops of lemon oil in a warm bath can refresh, energize, and invigorate a tender, aching body. Lemon oil stimulates and improves circulation and tones the blood vessels. The oil is especially helpful when massaged over broken capillaries or varicose veins.

Cosmetically, lemon oil is best for oily complexions, as it is a powerful astringent. For those with sensitive skin, lemon oil should first be diluted with a carrier oil. Add 3 to 5 drops lemon oil to 1 teaspoon sweet almond oil to produce a light blend that can be safely used to clear away a variety of skin imperfections. After applying this or other citrus essential oils to the skin, avoid sunlight for several hours. Many citrus oils contain a photosensitizing agent, increasing the skin's sensitivity to ultraviolet light.

Lemon essential oil has been a traditional treatment to lighten freckles. As it has both rejuvenating and lightening properties, lemon is also used to brighten dull skin. To create a refreshing and delightfully aromatic face brightener, add 6 drops each of lemon and lavender oil to 3 tablespoons pure distilled water. Gently spritz, splash, or use a clean cloth to apply the lemon water onto the face. Rub gently and follow with a moisturizer.

Because of its rousing and stimulating qualities, lemon has been considered a mild

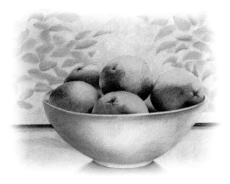

aphrodisiac and is associated with both Venus and Neptune, the planets of human and divine love. Its citrus fragrance uplifts not just the intellect, but also the heart. Lemon encourages the deep trust of love relationships, gently encouraging the heart to open by dispelling fear, especially of emotional entanglement. Lemon supports individuality while enhancing the joy of relationships. Lemon's inspiring, invigorating, and refreshing scent builds confidence, both in ourselves and in our interactions with the world.

GERM FIGHTER SPRAY

12 drops tea tree oil
6 drops eucalyptus oil
6 drops lemon oil
2 ounces distilled water or herbal tincture

Combine the ingredients and shake well to disperse the oils before each use. Dispense this formula from a spray bottle as needed on minor cuts, burns, or abrasions to prevent infection and speed healing. As an alternative to the distilled water, you can use a tincture made from an antiseptic herb such as Oregon grape root. If you do this, keep in mind that tinctures contain alcohol, which will make the essential oils disperse better and increase the antiseptic properties of the spray—but it will also sting more on an open wound. Apply immediately and then several times a day to keep the wound clean and encourage healing.

Uplifting Formula

6 drops bergamot oil
3 drops petitgrain oil
3 drops geranium oil
1 drop neroli (expensive, so optional)
2 ounces vegetable oil

Combine all the ingredients. Use as a massage oil, add
1 or 2 teaspoons to your bath, or add 1 teaspoon to a
foot bath. For an equally uplifting room or facial
spritzer, substitute the same amount of water for the
vegetable oil in this formula. Put the water formula in
a spray bottle and spritz or sniff throughout the day
as needed.

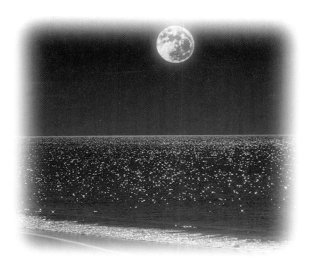

No pessimist ever discovered the secret of the stars,
or sailed to an uncharted land, or opened a new
heaven to the human spirit.

—HELEN KELLER

Life is a verb, not a noun.

—CHARLOTTE PERKINS GILMAN

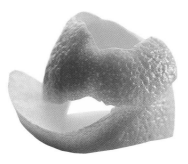

To me every hour of the light and dark is a miracle,

Every cubic inch of space is a miracle,

Every square yard of the surface of the earth is

spread with the same,

Every foot of the interior swarms with the same.

—WALT WHITMAN

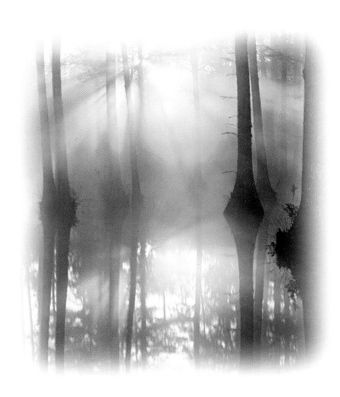

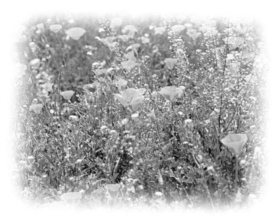

When one has much to put in them,

the day has a hundred pockets.

—FRIEDRICH NIETZSCHE

Spiderwebs, gossamer strands humming, are like hope—a strength that looks fragile, insignificant. Yet think what it does for the spider.

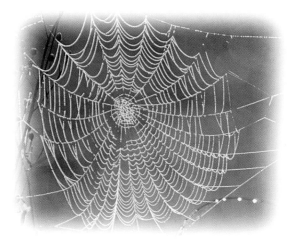

Life is mostly froth and bubble

Two things stand like stone,

Kindness in another's trouble,

Courage in your own.

—ADAM LINDSAY GORDON

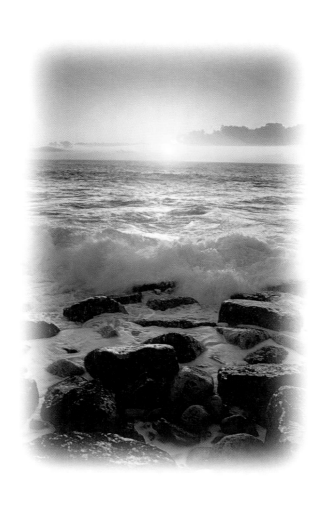

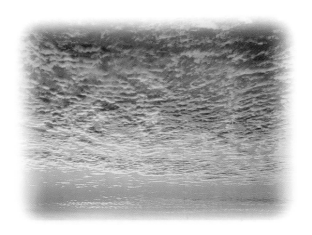

There are no days in life so memorable as those

which vibrated to some stroke of the imagination.

—RALPH WALDO EMERSON

Small as radiant grains of sand,

shooting stars blaze across the sky.

Like flaming rocks skipping across a black pond,

the meteors are faster than a thought,

swift as inspiration.

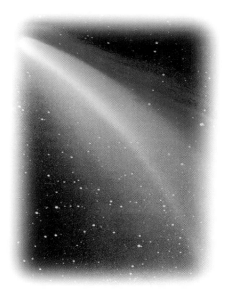

On this climb, I listen for the summit.

Above me, the rumble of thunder symphonies.

Below, adagios of melting snow.

Higher now: the sky hums

and with each note I scale upward.

Finally, atop this dizzy pinnacle

I sing my own, lone anthem, lungs bursting

with altitude and elation.

Echoed back, the hymn to myself

harmonizes with the music of the mountain.

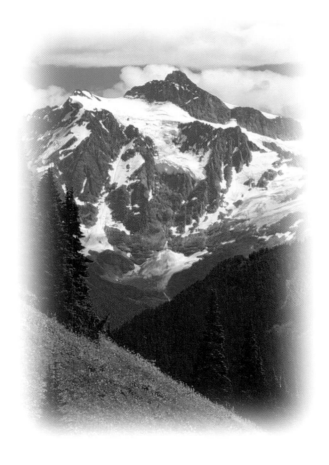

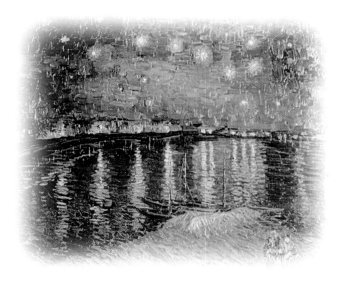

Without darkness, stars aren't visible.

Hope knows that clouds only cover the sun,

they don't banish it.

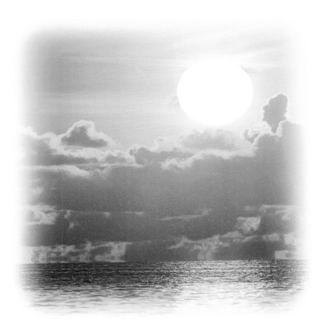

Summoned by dawn's warm caress,

sleepers glide awake and discover

dreams still in their hands,

treasures of nighttime mining.

No longer fossilized by weariness

and doubt like bugs in amber, they

skip into high-beam action like shafts of

light across a polished floor.

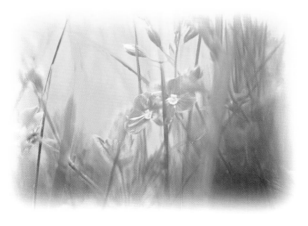

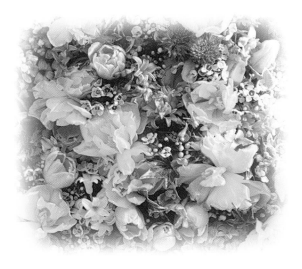

Real generosity toward the future lies in

giving all to the present.

—ALBERT CAMUS

I arise today

Through the strength of heaven,

Light of sun,

Radiance of moon,

Splendor of fire,

Speed of lightning,

Swiftness of wind

Depth of sea,

Stability of rock . . .

—SAINT PATRICK

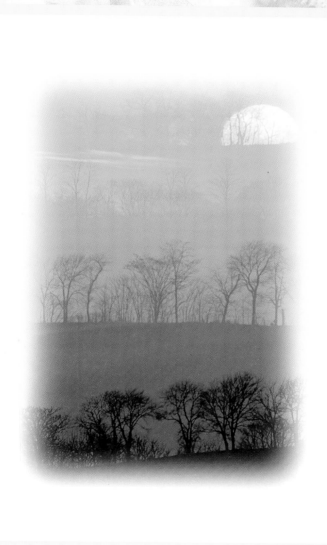

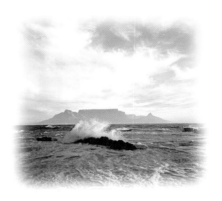

Look—the clouds are doing the rumba,

arcing their lithe arms over our heads!

Their wispy voices beckon to us below, calling:

"The sky is bright and cool!

Come, join our caper!

Let your body become frivolous."

After a day of cloud dancing,

we ground dwellers gloat with new bouyancy.

"Hope" is the thing with feathers—

That perches in the soul—

And sings the tune without the words—

And never stops—at all—

—EMILY DICKINSON

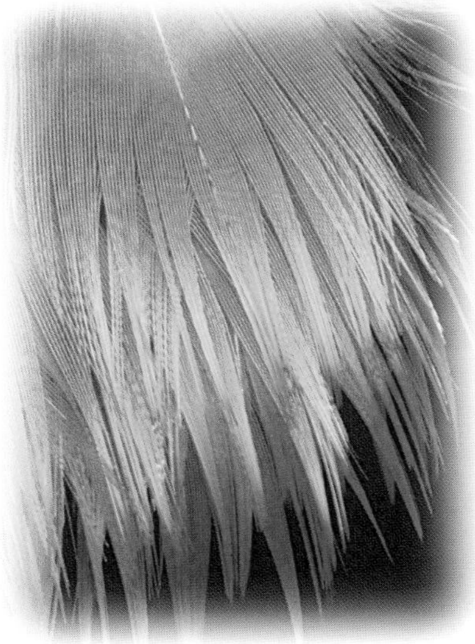

Open your eyes,

Dream but don't guess.

Your biggest surprise

Comes after Yes.

—MURIEL RUKEYSER

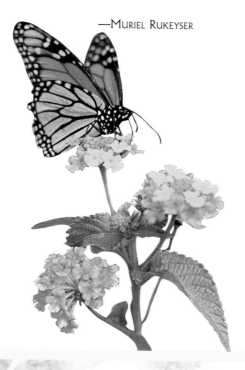

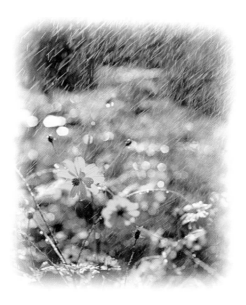

As flowers seek the sun from a sidewalk crack, we bloom in all seasons that would stunt our growing. For exultant, resilient, we accept the invitation to dance in summer's sweet breeze.

Come, come, whoever you are,

Wanderer, worshipper, lover of leaving,

it doesn't matter.

Ours is a caravan of endless joy . . .

—JELALUDDIN RUMI

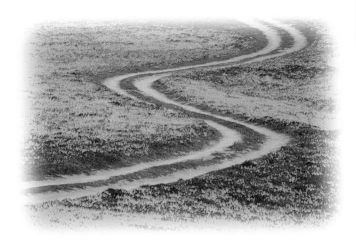

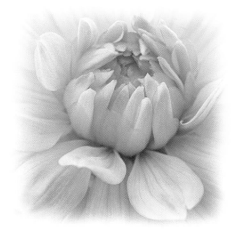

Keep your face to the sunshine and you cannot

see the shadow.

—HELEN KELLER

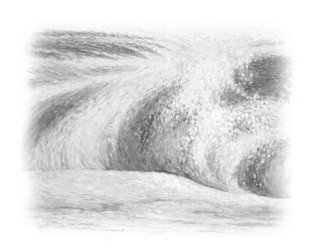

Energy is eternal delight.

—WILLIAM BLAKE

Give me the splendid silent sun with all

his beams full-dazzling,

Give me juicy autumnal fruit ripe and red

from the orchard,

Give me a field where the unmow'd grass grows,

Give me an arbor, give me the trellis'd grape ...

—WALT WHITMAN

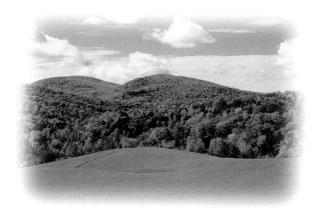

49

All our dreams can come true — if we have the courage to pursue them.

—FROM *GOD'S LITTLE INSTRUCTION BOOK FOR WOMEN*

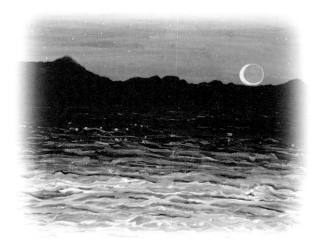

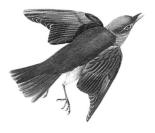

The bluebird carries the sky on his back.

—HENRY DAVID THOREAU

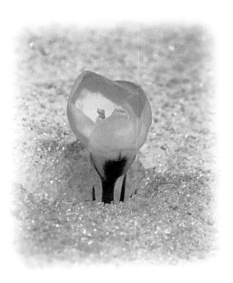

t is the seeker who finds crocuses blooming in the

snow and stars in the apple core;

the doubter who solves puzzles; and the stubborn,

like a butterfly beating its wings against a cocoon,

who emerges strong enough to fly.

i'd rather learn from one bird how to sing

than teach ten thousand stars how not to dance

—E.E. CUMMINGS

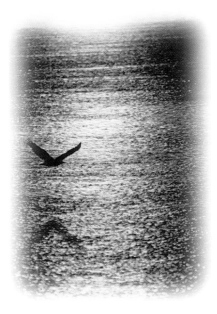

Take a daring, sailing leap

Knowing for one mid-air moment

childhood's splendid secrets,

The twirling kaleidoscope that is one ordinary day.

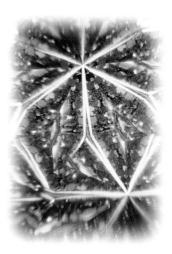

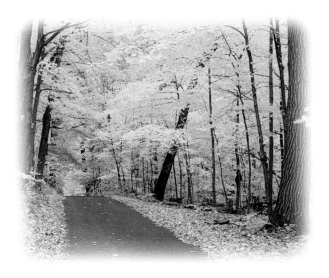

Alchemy is the burning belief that you can change whatever base metal exists in yourself and transform it slowly, gradually, and lovingly into gold.

You gain strength, courage, and confidence by every experience in which you really stop to look fear in the face ... You must do the thing you think you cannot do.

—Eleanor Roosevelt

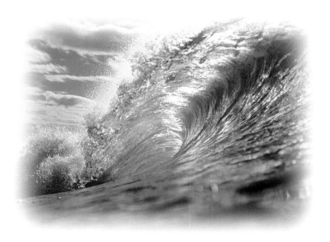

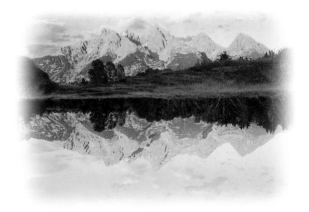

In the depths of winter, I finally learned that within

me there lay an invincible summer.

—ALBERT CAMUS

I am letting go of oatmeal mornings and having sunrises for breakfast. I am letting go of a sensible shoe life, donning ruby slippers, and finding a strut in my step. For all of my tomorrows, I'll lunch on sun rays and whisper good night to shooting stars.

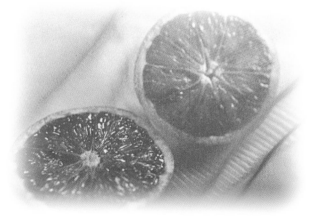

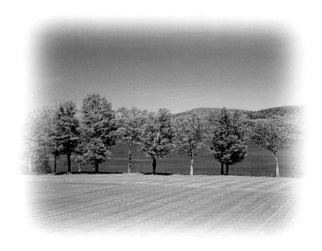

i thank you God for most this amazing

day: for the leaping greenly spirits of trees

and a blue true dream of sky; and for everything

which is natural which is infinite which is yes

—E.E. CUMMINGS

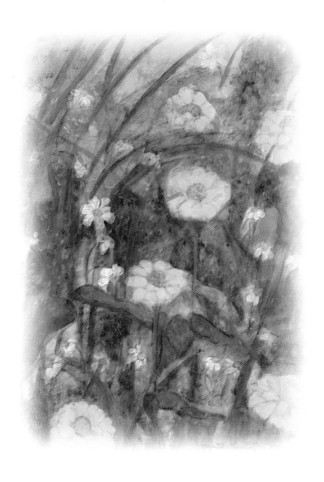